50 EASY CHAIR EXERCISES FOR SENIORS

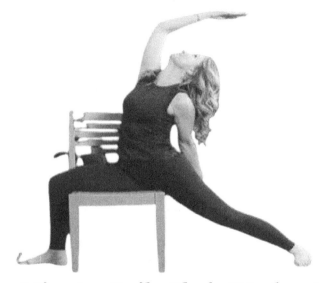

10 Minutes Daily Chair Workouts For Men and Woman To Lose Weight, Increase strength, Balance, Mobility and Flexibility

Christina J. Whitley

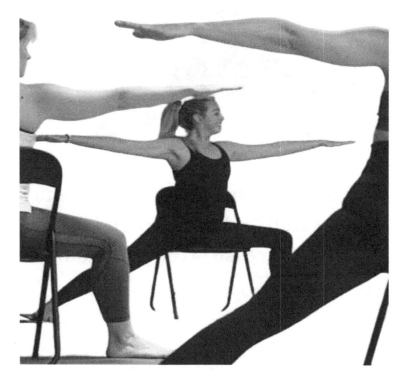

Table of contents

INTRODUCTION

The Transformation: Emily's Journey to a Stronger, More Vibrant Life

The seventy-one-year-old Emily had always valued her freedom and vigor. But as the years went by, her mobility, strength, flexibility, and balance started to decline, which made her increasingly frustrated. Even simple things like climbing stairs or bending to tie her shoelaces became difficult for her. Emily longed for a way to get back to her previous level of energy.

One day, Emily was browsing a local bookstore when she came upon a senior's guide on chair exercises. It promised to be her pass to renewed strength, mobility, flexibility, and balance. She made the decision to give it a shot and set off on a path that would transform her life.

The Discovery:

Emily discovered a wealth of exercises intended especially for seniors as she looked through the pages of the guide. The exercises focused on seated motions that she could modify to suit her own speed; they were mild yet effective. Emily was instantly enthralled with the notion that she could restore her vigor without having to dedicate herself to an intense exercise program.

Building Strength:

Emily started with the basics, embracing exercises like seated leg lifts and gentle resistance band workouts. She felt her leg muscles reawaken with each repetition, and soon, she noticed she could climb stairs with ease and stride confidently through her garden.

Regaining Flexibility:

Emily had once been a dancer, and she yearned to rediscover her flexibility. With the guidance of the exercises in the guide, she practiced gentle stretches and yoga-inspired movements. The range of motion in her joints expanded, and her body felt more limber than it had in years.

Balancing Act:

One of the guide's key strengths was its focus on balance. Emily practiced seated torso twists and heel-to-toe walking drills. These exercises gradually improved her balance and coordination. The sense of steadiness she regained brought back her confidence in navigating the world around her.

Freedom of Mobility:

The ultimate triumph for Emily was her renewed mobility. With increased strength, flexibility, and balance, her day-to-day life became more independent. She could walk through the park, bend to tie her shoelaces, and even explore hiking trails with her friends. She felt a newfound zest for life.

The Transformation:

The chair exercises guide had worked wonders, and Emily was living proof of its effectiveness. Her journey to increased strength, flexibility, balance, and mobility had rekindled her vitality and independence. She had discovered that age was no barrier to physical transformation, and the right exercises could provide a gateway to a vibrant and fulfilling life.

In the grand theater of life, the spotlight doesn't dim as the years advance. It's a stage where each of us plays a leading role, no matter our age. Yet, as we gracefully waltz through the years, our bodies may start to whisper hints of change, urging us to take action. And that's where our story begins, the story of discovering a renewed sense of strength, flexibility, balance, and mobility through 50 easy chair exercises crafted especially for seniors.

Aging, they say, is inevitable, but aging gracefully and actively is a choice. Whether you're looking to maintain your vitality, conquer new challenges, or simply relish the pleasures of daily life without aches and pains, this guide is your trusted companion. It's an invitation to embark on a journey that celebrates the wisdom of age, the power of experience, and the potential of every sunrise, no matter how many years it may bring.

Within these pages, you'll find a treasure trove of chair exercises thoughtfully designed for seniors—gentle, effective, and adaptable to various fitness levels. These exercises are not just routines; they are the keys to a more vibrant, active, and joyful life. They're your path to renewed strength, flexibility, balance, and mobility.

You might be wondering why chair exercises specifically? It's because the chair is more than a piece of furniture; it's a symbol of support, stability, and comfort. In this guide, the chair becomes your loyal companion, your training partner, and your trusty sidekick on the journey to a healthier, more resilient you.

So, let's embark on this journey together, embracing the gift of movement and the beauty of a life well-lived. It's time to defy expectations, to rise above limitations, and to shine in the spotlight, stronger, more flexible, balanced, and mobile than ever. It's time to script your own story of vitality, and these 50 easy chair exercises are the opening act.

CHAPTER 1

Why Chair Exercises Are Important for Seniors

Chair exercises offer an approach that is gentle, supportive, and adaptable to the needs and abilities of seniors. There are compelling reasons why chair exercises are important:

1. Improved Mobility: Seniors can experience easier and more enjoyable everyday activities by doing chair exercises to increase joint flexibility and mobility.

2. Muscle Strength: These exercises target various muscle groups, helping seniors maintain and build strength, which is crucial for balance and stability.

3. Cardiovascular Health: Chair exercises can get the heart pumping, promoting better circulation and heart health.

4. Pain Management: For those dealing with chronic pain or stiffness, chair exercises can provide relief and improve overall comfort.

5. Mental Well-Being: Staying physically active can boost mood, reduce stress, and support cognitive function.

6. Social Engagement: Chair exercises can be done individually or in group settings, fostering social connections and reducing feelings of isolation.

7. Safety and Accessibility: Chair exercises can be performed in the comfort of one's home or in community settings, and they are easily adaptable to individual fitness levels and needs.

How to Safely Perform Chair Exercises

The well-being of seniors is of paramount importance, and safety is a primary concern when engaging in any form of physical activity. To ensure a safe and enjoyable experience with chair exercises, it's imperative to consider the following:

1. Speak with a Healthcare Professional: It's a good idea to speak with a healthcare practitioner before starting a new fitness regimen, particularly if you have any underlying medical ailments or concerns.

2. Choose the Right Chair: Opt for a stable, armless chair with a firm seat, as it will provide the necessary support during exercises.

3. Warm-Up and Cool Down: Always begin with gentle warm-up exercises to prepare your body and finish with cooling-down stretches to prevent injury.

4. Proper Form and Technique: Pay close attention to your posture and movement during exercises to prevent strain or injury.

5. Listen to Your Body: Be attuned to your body's signals. If an exercise causes pain or discomfort, stop immediately and seek guidance.

6. Stay Hydrated: Drink water before, during, and after your chair exercise routine to prevent dehydration.

7. Consistency and Progression: Consistency is key. Gradually increase the duration and intensity of your exercises to continue reaping the benefits.

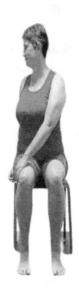

CHAPTER 2

Gentle Warm-Up Exercises

1. Seated Neck Rolls: Sit upright in your chair with your feet flat on the floor. Bring your ear near your shoulder as you slowly cock your head to one side. Gently roll your head forward, and then tilt your head to the other side. Complete this movement for 30 seconds, allowing your neck muscles to relax and release tension.

2. Shoulder Shrugs: Sit comfortably in your chair with your arms by your sides. Inhale deeply, and as you exhale, raise your shoulders up toward your ears in a shrugging motion. Hold for a moment, and then lower your shoulders as you inhale. Repeat this exercise for 20 seconds to relieve shoulder tension.

3. Ankle Circles: Sit with your feet firm on the ground. Lift one foot slightly off the ground and begin to make gentle circles with your ankle, first in a clockwise direction and then counterclockwise. Perform this exercise for 15 seconds on each ankle to improve ankle mobility and circulation.

4. Wrist Rotations: Extend your arms in front of you with your palms facing down. Begin by making small clockwise circles with your wrists for 15 seconds. Then, switch to counterclockwise circles for another 15 seconds. This exercise helps to warm up your wrists and improve flexibility.

5. Seated Torso Twist: Sit with your feet firm on the ground and your hands resting on your thighs. Inhale deeply, and as you exhale, twist your upper body to one side, reaching for the back of your chair with one hand and using the other to hold the armrest for support. After a little period of holding, move back to the middle. Repeat the twist on the other side. Perform this exercise for 30 seconds to gently warm up your spine and core.

These gentle warm-up exercises are designed to prepare your body for more vigorous chair exercises and help prevent injury by increasing blood flow, loosening muscles, and promoting flexibility.

CHAPTER 3

Upper Body Strength Exercises

1. Seated Arm Lifts: Place your feet firmly on the floor and sit with your back straight. Hold a light dumbbell or a water bottle in each hand. Start with your arms at your sides. Slowly lift both arms to shoulder height, then lower them back down. Perform 3 sets of 12-15 reps to strengthen your shoulders and upper arms.

2. Seated Bicep Curls: Sit with your back straight, holding a dumbbell or water bottle in each hand, palms facing forward. Keep your elbows close to your sides as you curl the weights upward, then lower them back down. Do 3 sets of 12-15 reps to target your biceps.

3. Overhead Press: Sit with your back straight, holding a dumbbell or a water bottle in each hand. Bend your elbows at a 90-degree angle. Press the weights overhead until your arms are fully extended, then lower them back down. Perform 3 sets of 10-12 reps to work on your shoulder strength.

4. Chest Squeezes: Place your feet firmly on the floor and sit with your back straight. Hold a soft ball or a cushion in front of your chest with both hands. Squeeze the ball as hard as you can for 5 seconds, then release. Repeat for 3 sets of 10 squeezes to strengthen your chest and improve arm coordination.

5. Tricep Dips: Scoot to the edge of your chair with your hands on the edge of the seat, fingers pointing forward. Slide your hips off the chair while keeping your feet flat on the ground. Bend your elbows, lowering your body, then straighten your arms to raise yourself back up. Do 3 sets of 10-12 reps to target your triceps and build upper body strength.

These upper body strength exercises are designed to help seniors build and maintain muscle strength in the arms, shoulders, and chest, which can improve daily activities and enhance overall well-being.

CHAPTER 4

Lower Body Strength Exercises

1. Seated Leg Extensions: Maintain a straight back when you sit at the edge of your chair. Raise one leg straight up off the ground and place it in front of you. After holding it for a short while, bring it back down. Do 3 sets of 12-15 reps for each leg to strengthen your quadriceps.

2. Seated Leg Lifts: While seated, extend one leg straight out in front of you and lift it as high as you comfortably can. Lower it back down and repeat for 3 sets of 10-12 reps for each leg. This exercise targets your hip flexors and thighs.

3. Seated Marching: Sit with your feet firm on the ground. Lift one knee as high as possible and then lower it, alternating between legs as if you are marching in place. Perform this exercise for 1-2 minutes to improve leg strength and coordination.

4. Seated Heel Raises: Sit with your feet firm on the ground. While maintaining the balls of your feet on the ground, raise your heels as high as you can. Lower your heels back down and repeat for 3 sets of 12-15 reps to work on your calf muscles.

5. Seated Squats: Position yourself at the chair's edge, keeping your feet shoulder-width apart. Stand up from the chair and then lower yourself back down, almost sitting, but not quite. Do 3 sets of 10-12 reps to strengthen your quadriceps, hamstrings, and glutes.

These lower body strength exercises are designed to help seniors improve muscle strength in their legs, which is essential for maintaining balance, stability, and mobility in daily life.

CHAPTER 5

Balance and Flexibility Exercises

1. Seated Twists: Sit with your feet on the ground and your hands on your thighs. Slowly twist your upper body to one side while keeping your hips facing forward. Hold the twist for a few seconds, then return to the center and repeat on the other side. Do 3 sets of 10-12 twists to improve spinal flexibility and balance.

2. Seated Side Leg Lifts: Sit with your back firm and your feet on the ground. Lift one leg out to the side as high as you comfortably can, then lower it back down. Perform 3 sets of 12-15 lifts for each leg to enhance hip flexibility and strengthen the abductor muscles.

3. Seated Hip Circles: Sit with your feet on the ground and your hands on your hips. Slowly circle your hips clockwise for 15 seconds and then counterclockwise for another 15 seconds. This exercise improves hip mobility and flexibility.

4. Seated Toe Touches: Sit with your legs extended in front of you. Reach your arms toward your toes while keeping your back straight. Hold the stretch for 15-30 seconds. Perform 3 sets of 10-12 stretches to enhance hamstring and lower back flexibility.

5. Seated Butterfly Stretch: Place your feet firmly on the floor and sit with your back straight. Bring the soles of your feet together and let your knees gently fall out to the sides. Hold your feet with your hands and gently press down on your knees to feel the stretch in your inner thighs. Hold for 20-30 seconds and release. This exercise improves hip and groin flexibility.

These balance and flexibility exercises are designed to help seniors maintain and improve their range of motion and balance, reducing the risk of falls and enhancing overall mobility.

CHAPTER 6

Cardiovascular Chair Exercises

1. Seated High Knees: Maintain a straight back when you sit at the edge of your chair. Lift one knee as high as you can, then quickly switch to the other knee. Continue this movement, resembling a marching motion, for 1-2 minutes. This exercise raises your heart rate and improves circulation.

2. Seated Marching in Place: Sit with your feet firm on the floor. Lift your knees as high as you can while "marching" in place for 2-3 minutes. This exercise provides a low-impact way to get your heart pumping.

3. Seated Jumping Jacks: Sit with your feet together. As you spread your arms out to the sides, simultaneously jump your feet apart. Then, bring your arms and legs back to the starting position. Perform this seated jumping jack motion for 1-2 minutes to boost your cardiovascular fitness.

4. Seated Knee Taps: Sit with your feet firm on the ground and your arms at your sides. Rapidly tap your knees with your hands while keeping your back straight. Continue this motion for 2-3 minutes to elevate your heart rate and promote circulation.

5. Seated Leg Crosses: Sit with your feet firm on the floor. Raise one leg and cross it over the other, alternating between legs at a brisk pace. Do this exercise for 2-3 minutes to increase your heart rate and work on leg strength and flexibility.

These cardiovascular chair exercises are designed to help seniors improve their heart health and endurance in a seated position, making them an excellent option for those with limited mobility or balance concerns.

CHAPTER 7

Core and Posture Exercises

1. Seated Torso Twists: Sit with your feet firm on the ground and your hands on your thighs. Inhale deeply, and as you exhale, twist your upper body to one side, reaching for the back of your chair with one hand and using the other to hold the armrest for support. Hold the twist for a few seconds, then return to the center and repeat on the other side. Perform this exercise for 3 sets of 10-12 twists to improve core strength and spinal flexibility.

2. Seated Abdominal Contractions: Sit with your feet firm on the ground and your back straight. Inhale deeply, and as you exhale, contract your abdominal muscles, pulling your navel toward your spine. Hold the contraction for a few seconds, then release. Repeat for 3 sets of 15-20 contractions to strengthen your core.

3. Seated Back Stretches: Sit with your feet firm on the ground and your hands on your hips. Gently arch your back, pushing your chest forward while looking up. Hold the stretch for 15-20 seconds. Then, round your back, bringing your chin toward your chest. Hold this stretch for another 15-20 seconds. This exercise helps improve posture and flexibility in the spine.

4. Seated Pelvic Tilts: Sit with your feet firm on the ground and your hands on your thighs. Inhale deeply, and as you exhale, tilt your pelvis forward, arching your lower back. Inhale and tilt your pelvis backward, rounding your lower back. Perform this tilting motion for 3 sets of 10-12 repetitions to enhance pelvic and lower back flexibility and strengthen your core.

5. Seated Cat-Cow Stretch: Sit with your feet firm on the ground and your hands on your thighs. Inhale deeply and arch your back, pushing your chest forward while looking up (the "cow" position). Then, exhale and round your back, bringing your chin to your chest (the "cat" position). Repeat this cat-cow stretch for 3 sets of 10-12 repetitions to improve spine flexibility and posture.

These core and posture exercises are designed to help seniors strengthen their core muscles, which are essential for maintaining proper posture and spinal health. They also aid in reducing the risk of back pain and enhancing overall stability.

CHAPTER 8

Relaxation and Breathing Exercises

1. Seated Deep Breathing: Sit with your back straight and your feet firm on the ground. Close your eyes and take a slow, deep breath in through your nose, allowing your abdomen to rise as you fill your lungs. Exhale slowly through your mouth. Repeat this deep breathing for 3-5 minutes to promote relaxation and reduce stress.

2. Seated Shoulder Rolls: Sit with your back straight and your hands resting on your thighs. Inhale deeply, and as you exhale, roll your shoulders forward in a circular motion. Inhale and roll your shoulders backward. Repeat this shoulder roll for 1-2 minutes to release tension in your shoulder and neck muscles.

3. Seated Neck Stretches: Sit with your feet firm on the ground and your hands on your thighs. Gently tilt your head to one side, bringing your ear toward your shoulder. Hold the stretch for 15-20 seconds, then switch to the other side. Perform this neck stretch to relieve tension in the neck and promote relaxation.

4. Seated Meditation: Find a comfortable and quiet place to sit in your chair. Close your eyes and focus on your breath.

Inhale and exhale naturally, paying attention to the rhythm of your breath. Clear your mind and let go of any stress or worries. Meditate for 5-10 minutes to promote mental relaxation and mindfulness.

5. Seated Shoulder Stretch: Sit with your feet firm on the ground and interlace your fingers in front of you. Inhale deeply, and as you exhale, push your palms away from your body while rounding your back. Hold the stretch for 15-20 seconds. Release and repeat 2-3 times to relieve tension in your shoulders and upper back.

These relaxation and breathing exercises are designed to help seniors reduce stress, enhance relaxation, and achieve a sense of inner calm. Practicing these exercises regularly can have a positive impact on overall well-being and mental health.

CHAPTER 9

Fun and Functional Exercises

1. Seated Soccer Ball Kicks: Position yourself at the edge of the chair, keeping your feet flat on the ground and your back straight. Place a small, soft ball between your feet. Kick the ball back and forth with your feet, as if you're playing a game of seated soccer. This exercise improves lower body coordination and can be a fun way to stay active.

2. Seated Basketball Shoots: Sit with your feet firm on the ground and hold a soft ball in your hands. Pretend you're shooting hoops by extending your arms upward and "shooting" the ball into an imaginary basket. Repeat this motion for 2-3 minutes to enhance hand-eye coordination and upper body strength.

3. Seated Hula Hoop: Sit with your feet firm on the ground and hold a hula hoop in your hands. Make circular motions with the hoop, imitating the action of hula hooping. This exercise improves arm and shoulder mobility while adding a playful element to your routine.

4. Seated Dance Moves: Put on some music you enjoy and simply dance in your chair. Move your upper body, tap your feet, and have fun with it. Dancing is a fantastic way to improve overall body coordination, flexibility, and mood.

5. **Seated Balloon Volleyball:** Find a partner or group of friends, and sit across from each other with a balloon placed in the middle. Use your hands to keep the balloon from touching the ground, volleying it back and forth. This exercise is a social, enjoyable way to improve upper body coordination and teamwork.

These fun and functional exercises are designed to not only help seniors stay active but also to add an element of enjoyment to their fitness routine. They encourage social interaction, physical activity, and a sense of playfulness.

CHAPTER 10

Partner and Group Exercises

1. Chair Yoga for Two: Partner up with another person and sit facing each other in chairs. Follow a chair yoga routine together, moving through gentle stretches and poses while mirroring each other's movements. This exercise enhances flexibility, balance, and provides a sense of connection.

2. Chair Exercise Bingo: Create a bingo card with various chair exercises listed in each square. Partner up or form a group and take turns calling out an exercise for everyone to perform. Participants mark off exercises on their cards as they complete them. The first one to get a row or column marked wins a prize.

3. Chair Exercise Relay: Set up an exercise relay course in a group setting. Create stations with different chair exercises, and participants take turns moving from one station to the next. For example, one station could be chair squats, the next could be seated leg lifts, and so on. This exercise promotes teamwork, coordination, and cardiovascular fitness.

4. Chair Exercise Social Hour: Organize a group session where everyone can gather to chat, enjoy refreshments, and engage in seated exercises. An instructor can lead the group through a series of chair exercises designed for all fitness levels while participants socialize. This exercise encourages social interaction and overall well-being.

5. Chair Dance Party: Put on some music and have a dance party with a partner or in a group of friends. In your chairs, dance to the rhythm and enjoy moving to the beat. This exercise is not only fun but also promotes cardiovascular health, coordination, and a sense of community.

These partner and group exercises are designed to foster social connections, add an element of fun to fitness routines, and create a supportive environment for seniors to stay active and engaged.

CHAPTER 11

Cool Down and Stretching Exercises

1. Seated Quad Stretches: Sit with your feet firm on the ground. Bend one knee and bring your heel toward your buttocks. Gently grasp your ankle and pull it closer to your glutes. Hold the stretch for 15-20 seconds for each leg to relieve tension in the quadriceps.

2. Seated Hamstring Stretches: Sit with your feet firm on the ground and extend one leg straight out in front of you. Reach for your toes with both hands while keeping your back straight. Hold the stretch for 15-20 seconds for each leg to improve hamstring flexibility.

3. Seated Chest Opener: Sit with your feet firm on the ground and clasp your hands behind your back. Straighten your arms and gently lift them away from your back while squeezing your shoulder blades together. This stretch helps open the chest and improve posture. Hold for 15-20 seconds.

4. Seated Full Body Stretch: Sit with your feet firm on the ground and extend your arms overhead. Reach up and elongate your body as much as possible. Hold the stretch for 20-30 seconds to relieve tension and promote full-body flexibility.

5. Seated Relaxation Breathing: After a series of stretches, sit comfortably in your chair with your eyes closed. Take slow, deep breaths in through your nose and exhale through your mouth. As you breathe out, focus on releasing any remaining tension in your body. Spend 2-3 minutes in this relaxed, deep-breathing state.

These cool down and stretching exercises are essential for seniors to improve flexibility, prevent muscle soreness, and maintain overall mobility. They provide a gentle way to end a chair exercise routine and promote relaxation.

CHAPTER 12

Using Props and Accessories

Incorporating props and accessories into chair exercises can greatly enhance the effectiveness, variety, and overall enjoyment of your fitness routine, especially for seniors. These additions introduce new elements to your workout, making it more engaging and challenging. Here's a closer look at how props and accessories can be beneficial:

1. Resistance Bands: A fantastic item for adding resistance to your chair exercises is an elastic resistance band. They are appropriate for a range of fitness levels because they are available in different resistance levels. Resistance bands can be used in exercises like seated bicep curls, leg lifts, and chest squeezes to target particular muscular areas, such as the arms, legs, and chest. These bands provide a mild yet effective resistance that aids in muscle toning and strengthening.

2. Soft Balls: Soft, lightweight balls are versatile props that can be used for various exercises. They are ideal for improving hand-eye coordination and targeting core muscles. For instance, you can hold a soft ball while doing seated twists, passing it between your hands to engage your core and upper body. Additionally, you can use the ball for gentle arm and leg exercises, enhancing balance and flexibility.

3. Small Hand Weights: For seniors looking to increase the intensity of their chair exercises, small hand weights are a valuable addition. They can be held during arm exercises like overhead presses or used to add weight to leg lifts. These weights help build upper body strength and muscle tone. It's important to start with light weights and gradually increase the resistance as you become more comfortable with the exercises.

4. Stretch Bands: Stretch bands with handles provide a convenient way to perform various upper body exercises while seated. You can use them for seated rows, chest presses, and tricep extensions. These bands offer resistance, which can help seniors develop and maintain upper body strength.

5. Yoga Straps: Yoga straps can assist in stretching and flexibility exercises. They are particularly useful for individuals with limited flexibility. By using a yoga strap, you can perform leg stretches and deepening stretches for the upper body with added support. These straps ensure that you can safely and effectively engage in stretching routines, promoting better overall flexibility.

6. Balance Cushions: Adding a balance cushion or wobble cushion to your chair exercises can enhance your core stability and balance. Simply place it on your chair to create an unstable surface. This forces your core muscles to engage as you sit, helping you develop better balance and stability over time.

Incorporating these props and accessories into your chair exercise routine can offer a wide range of benefits, including increased strength, improved flexibility, enhanced balance, and a more engaging exercise experience. Remember to start with lighter resistance levels or props to ensure safety, and gradually progress as you become more comfortable and confident with your chair exercises.

Chair Safety Guidelines

Chair exercises are a valuable and accessible way for seniors to maintain their fitness, but safety should always be a top priority. Following chair safety guidelines is essential to prevent injuries and ensure a comfortable and effective workout. Here are important chair safety tips for seniors:

1. Chair Selection: Choose a stable, sturdy chair with a firm seat. Avoid chairs with wheels or swivel bases, as they can be unstable for exercising. The chair should have armrests for support, especially during balance exercises.

2. Proper Seating: Sit with your back straight against the backrest of the chair. Your feet should be flat on the floor, hip-width apart. This position provides stability and support during exercises.

3. Warm-Up and Cool Down: Always start your chair exercise routine with a gentle warm-up to prepare your muscles and end with a cool down to help your body recover. Warm-up and cool-down exercises are essential for preventing strains and injuries.

4. Proper Form and Technique: Pay close attention to your posture and movement during exercises. Keep your movements controlled and precise to avoid overextending or straining your muscles. If you're unsure about the correct form, consider working with a qualified instructor.

5. Listen to Your Body: Be mindful of how your body feels during exercises. If you experience pain, discomfort, or dizziness, stop the exercise immediately. It's essential to prioritize your safety and comfort.

6. Consult with a Healthcare Professional: Before starting a new exercise routine, especially if you have underlying health conditions, consult with your healthcare provider. They can provide guidance on the types of exercises that are safe and appropriate for your specific needs.

7. Stay Hydrated: Drink water before, during, and after your chair exercise routine to stay hydrated. Dehydration can lead to fatigue and increase the risk of injury, so it's crucial to maintain proper hydration.

8. Appropriate Footwear: Wear comfortable and supportive shoes with non-slip soles. Good footwear helps with balance and stability during exercises.

9. Gradual Progression: Start with exercises that match your current fitness level. Gradually increase the duration and intensity of your workouts as your strength and confidence grow. Avoid overexertion, especially if you're just beginning an exercise routine.

10. Safety Rails or Handles: If available, consider adding safety rails or handles to your chair or exercise area. These can provide additional support during balance exercises.

11. Clear Exercise Space: Ensure that your exercise area is clear of obstacles and tripping hazards. Create a safe and clutter-free environment to reduce the risk of accidents.

12. Use Props Carefully: If you incorporate props like resistance bands or hand weights, make sure you use them with caution. Start with light resistance levels and focus on proper technique to avoid strains or injuries.

By adhering to these chair safety guidelines, seniors can enjoy the many benefits of chair exercises while minimizing the risk of accidents and injuries. Safety is a critical component of any fitness routine, and it allows seniors to stay active with confidence and peace of mind.

CHAPTER 13

Testimonials and Success Stories

Real-Life Stories of Improved Health and Well-Being

In this chapter, we celebrate the real-life success stories of seniors who have embraced chair exercises and experienced remarkable improvements in their health and well-being. These inspirational stories illustrate the transformative power of chair exercises and how they have positively impacted the lives of older adults. We hope these stories serve as motivation for you to embark on your own chair exercise journey and discover the incredible benefits for yourself.

Irene's Journey to Mobility

Irene, at the age of 70, found herself struggling with mobility issues due to arthritis. She could no longer enjoy her daily walks or easily perform everyday tasks. Determined to regain her independence, she began a chair exercise routine that focused on improving her leg strength. With dedication and time, Irene regained the ability to walk without assistance and now enjoys her daily strolls in the park, pain-free.

Fred's Heartfelt Transformation

After experiencing a heart attack, Fred, aged 75, was determined to improve his cardiovascular health. He started incorporating chair exercises that targeted his heart health, such as seated jumping jacks and seated high knees. Over time, Fred's energy levels increased, his blood pressure dropped, and he could perform his daily activities without feeling fatigued.

Grace's Journey to Posture Perfection

At 80 years young, Grace struggled with poor posture and lower back pain. She incorporated chair exercises that focused on core strength and posture improvement. Within months, Grace noticed a significant change in her posture and a reduction in her back pain. Now she stands taller, walks with confidence, and participates in activities she once thought were beyond her reach.

Robert's Tale of Weight Management

Robert, at the age of 68, faced challenges with his weight. He embraced chair exercises as part of his daily routine to help with weight management. With exercises like seated squats and chair marches, Robert not only shed unwanted pounds but also gained strength and muscle tone. His journey is a testament to the effectiveness of chair exercises in achieving fitness goals.

Judy's Inspiration for Seniors Everywhere

Judy, a vibrant 85-year-old, embodies the spirit of chair exercises and shares her wisdom with other seniors. Through her dedication to seated yoga and stretching, Judy remains flexible, agile, and full of life. She encourages seniors everywhere to make chair exercises a part of their daily routine, emphasizing that it's never too late to start a fitness journey.

These real-life stories showcase the incredible potential of chair exercises to enhance the health and well-being of seniors. Through commitment, perseverance, and the right chair exercise routine, remarkable transformations are possible. The words and experiences of these individuals serve as inspiration for all seniors to embrace chair exercises and enjoy the myriad benefits they offer. Whether you're looking to regain mobility, improve heart health, perfect your posture, manage weight, or simply lead a more active and fulfilling life, chair exercises can be your pathway to success.

CONCLUSION

The Lifelong Benefits of Chair Exercises for Seniors

In the journey through the pages of this guide, we've explored the world of chair exercises and their profound impact on the health and well-being of seniors. We've witnessed the transformative power of these gentle yet effective routines that can be tailored to every fitness level and mobility. Now, as we conclude our exploration, let's reflect on the lifelong benefits that chair exercises offer to seniors.

Chair exercises provide seniors with a path to improved mobility and flexibility, making everyday activities more manageable and enjoyable. These routines help seniors regain ease of movement, whether it's walking, bending, or reaching. Moreover, they contribute to enhanced muscle strength and tone, which is crucial for functional independence and preventing age-related muscle loss.

Enhanced cardiovascular health is another significant advantage of chair exercises. These routines gently elevate the heart rate, improving circulation, lowering blood pressure, and strengthening the heart. Seniors can experience better cardiovascular health without subjecting themselves to high-impact exercises.

Chair exercises focus on posture and balance, offering seniors the chance to improve their stability and reduce the risk of falls. This benefit extends to better posture, which has aesthetic and functional advantages, contributing to an overall sense of well-being.

For seniors interested in weight management, chair exercises are a valuable tool. They facilitate calorie burning, weight maintenance, and obesity-related health management. It's a holistic approach to maintaining a healthy weight.

The mental benefits of chair exercises are equally important. Regular physical activity reduces stress, enhances mood, and improves cognitive function. Seniors can maintain a positive outlook and reduce the risk of depression and anxiety by incorporating these exercises into their routines.

Finally, chair exercises offer a sense of social engagement. Seniors can come together, share their experiences, and enjoy the camaraderie of like-minded individuals. This community support adds a vital dimension to overall well-being.

In conclusion, chair exercises provide seniors with a lifeline to a more fulfilling and active life. With dedication and a commitment to personal health, seniors can realize the profound and lifelong benefits of these exercises. This guide has served as a resource and an inspiration for seniors to take the first step on the path to better health, a more vibrant life, and an enduring sense of well-being.

We encourage you to embrace chair exercises as a valuable and sustainable component of your daily routine. The benefits are lifelong, the journey is rewarding, and the time to start is now. Here's to a healthier, happier, and more active life through the power of chair exercises.

FITNESS

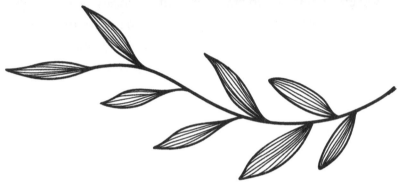

PLANNER

Fitness Planner

NAME:

DATE:

BREAKFAST

LUNCH

DINNER

SNACK

EXERCISE

SET   REP   NOTES

Fitness Planner

NAME: **DATE:**

BREAKFAST   LUNCH

DINNER   SNACK

EXERCISE   SET   REP   NOTES

Fitness Planner

NAME: **DATE:**

BREAKFAST   LUNCH

DINNER   SNACK

EXERCISE	SET	REP	NOTES

Fitness
Planner

NAME: **DATE:**

BREAKFAST   ### LUNCH

DINNER   ### SNACK

EXERCISE   SET   REP   NOTES

Fitness Planner

NAME:　　　　　**DATE:**

BREAKFAST

LUNCH

DINNER

SNACK

EXERCISE	SET	REP	NOTES

Fitness Planner

NAME: **DATE:**

BREAKFAST   LUNCH

DINNER   SNACK

EXERCISE   SET   REP   NOTES

Fitness Planner

NAME:

DATE:

BREAKFAST

LUNCH

DINNER

SNACK

EXERCISE

EXERCISE	SET	REP	NOTES

Fitness
Planner

NAME: DATE:

BREAKFAST   LUNCH

DINNER   SNACK

EXERCISE   SET   REP   NOTES

Fitness Planner

NAME: **DATE:**

BREAKFAST

LUNCH

DINNER

SNACK

EXERCISE	SET	REP	NOTES

Fitness Planner

NAME: **DATE:**

BREAKFAST   ### LUNCH

DINNER   ### SNACK

EXERCISE   SET   REP   NOTES

Made in the USA
Las Vegas, NV
29 November 2023

81803862R00036